I0842452

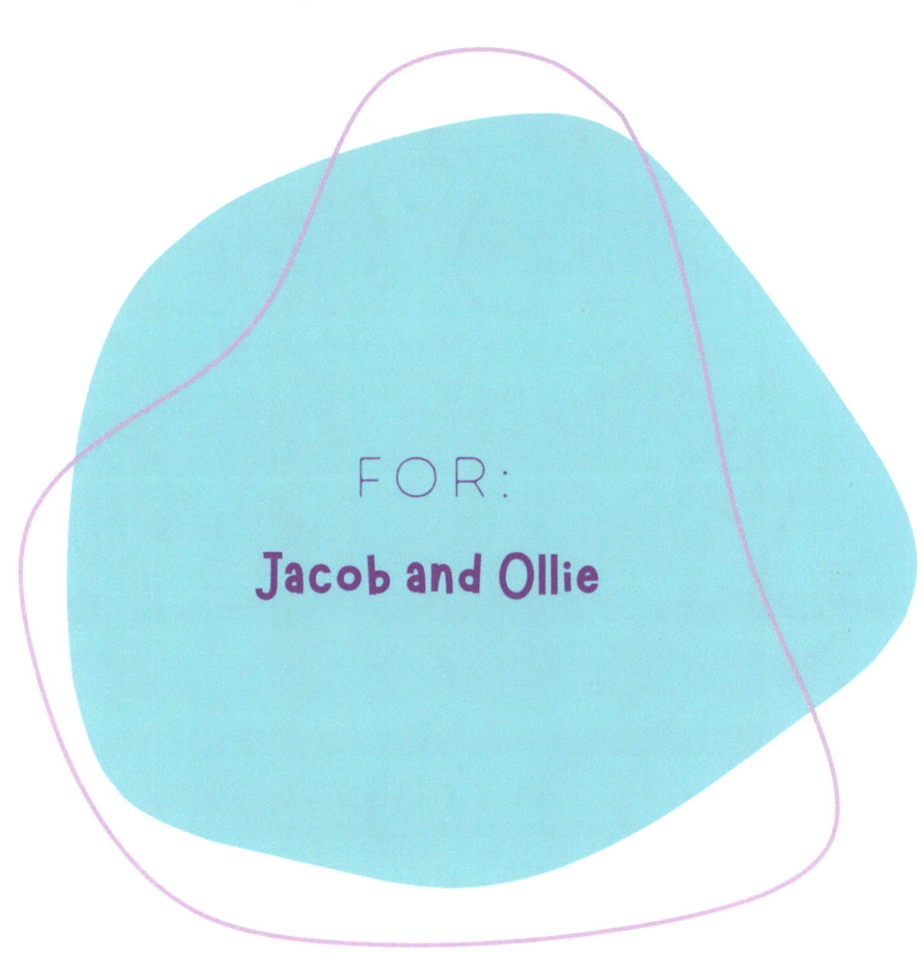

FOR:
Jacob and Ollie

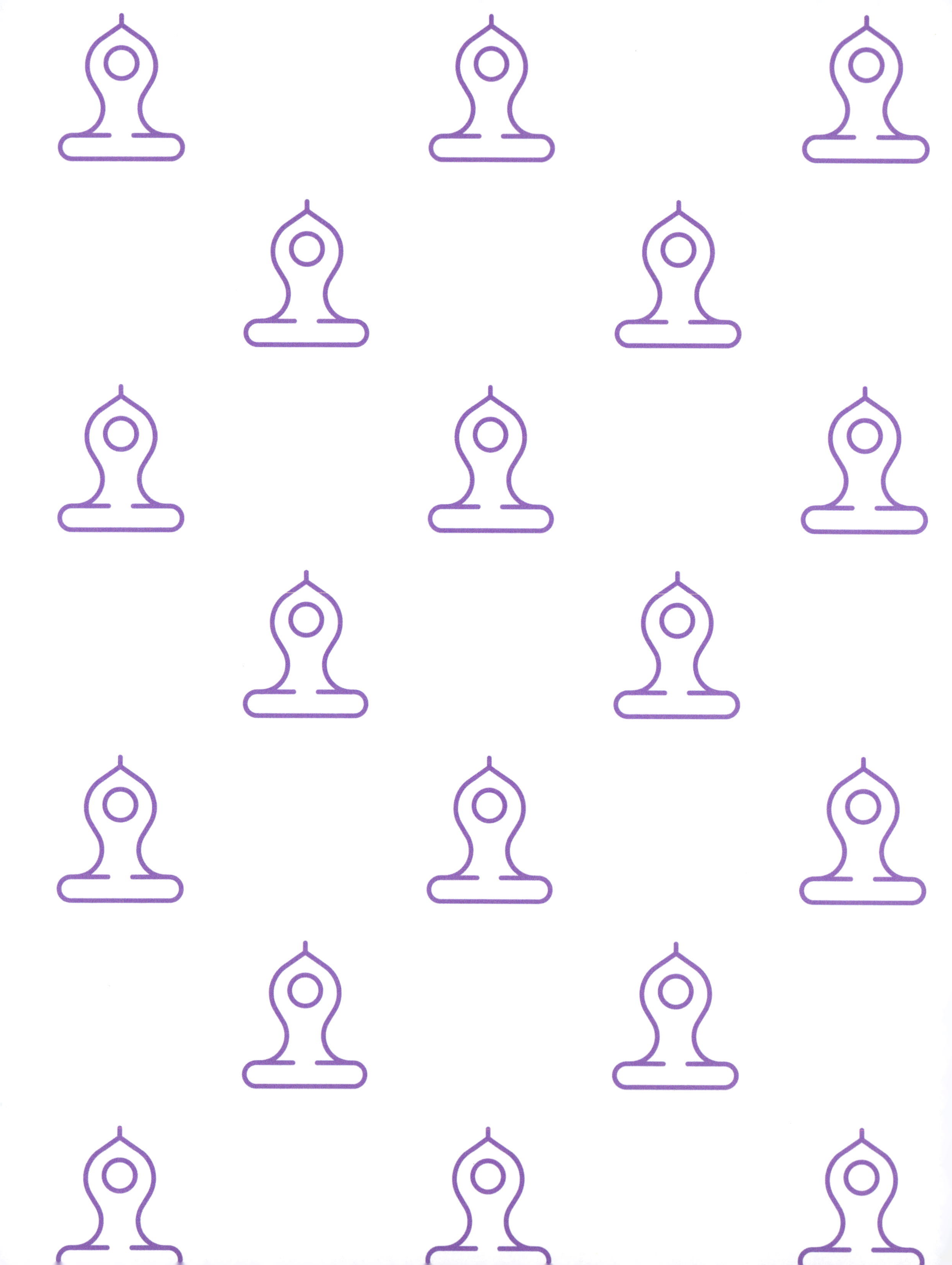

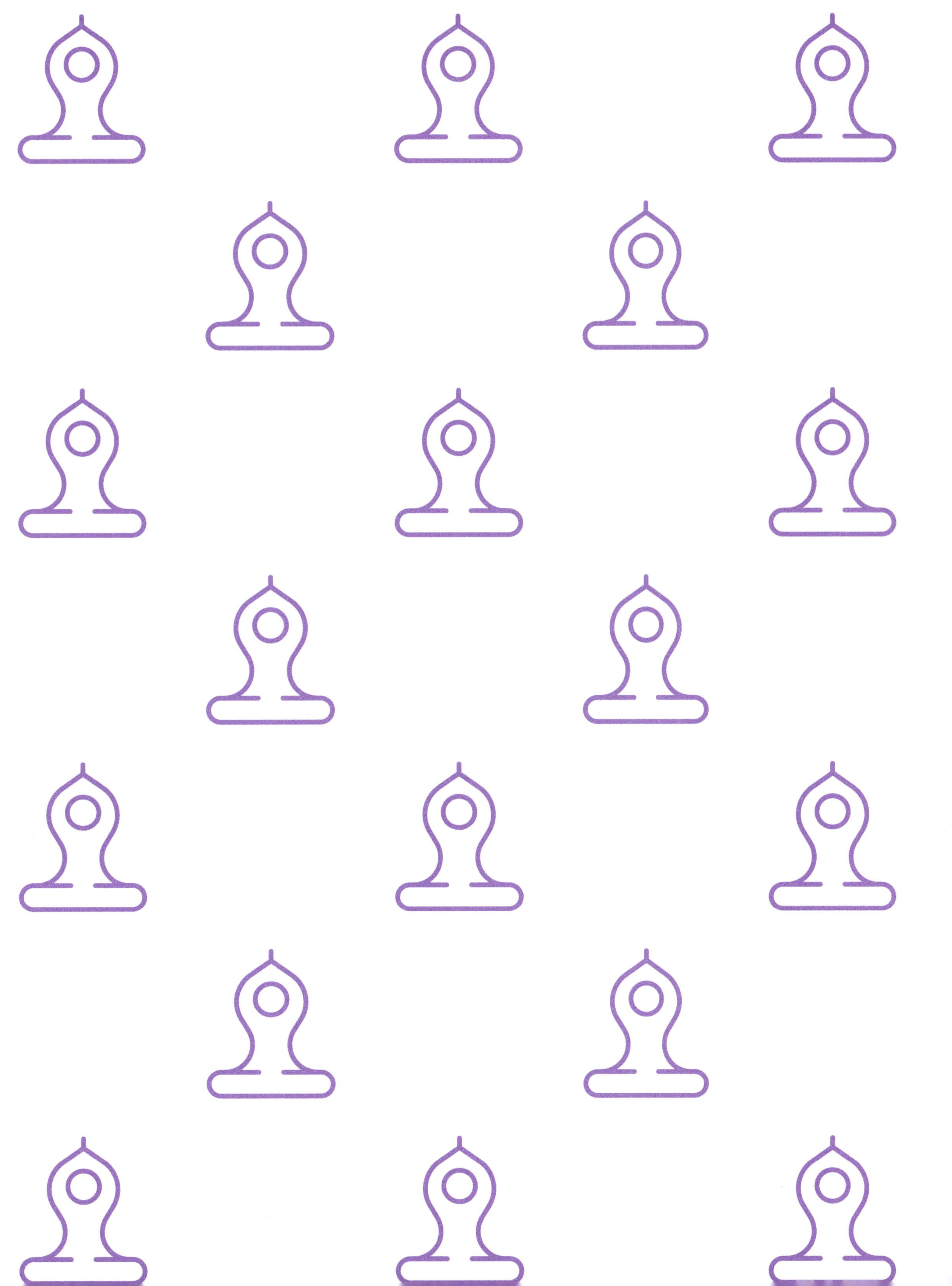

LITTLE YOGIS

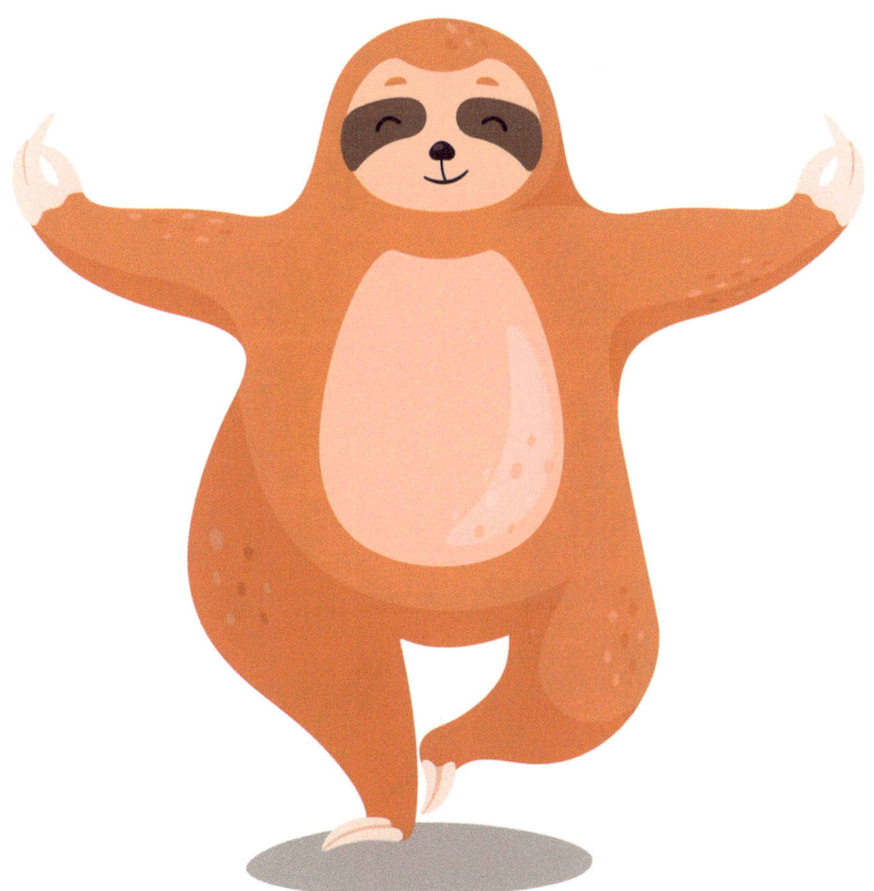

YOGA POSES FOR KIDS

THIS BOOK BELONGS TO:

. . . .

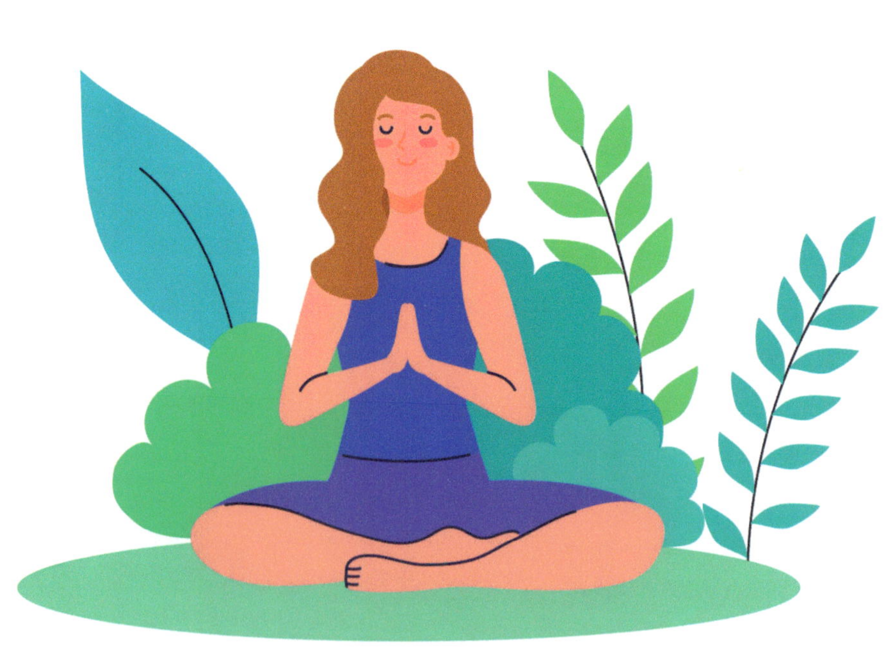

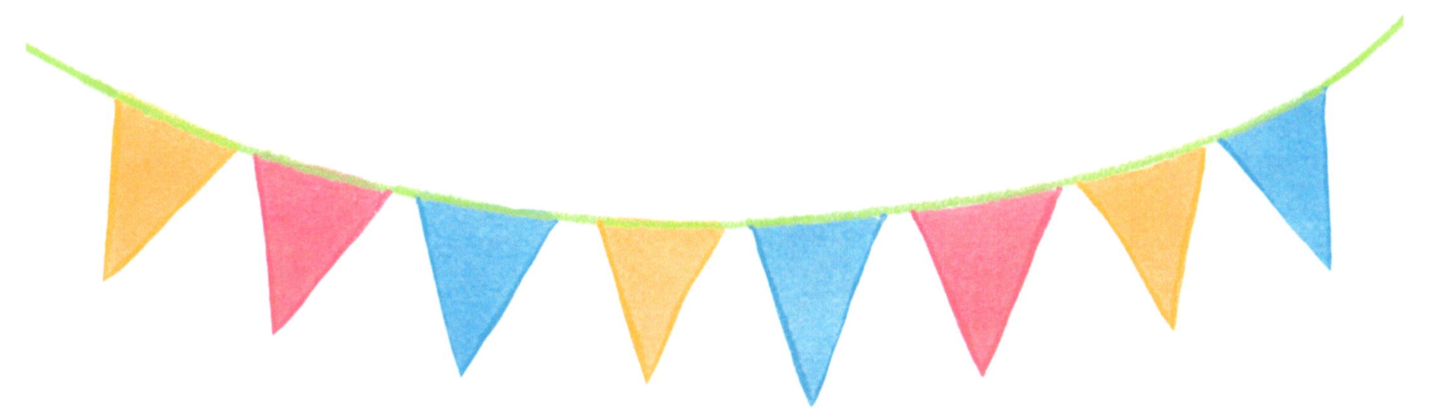

LET'S GET
STARTED

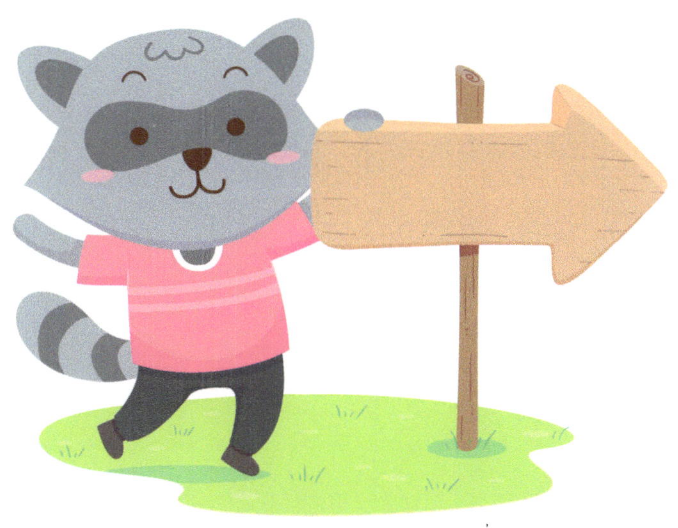

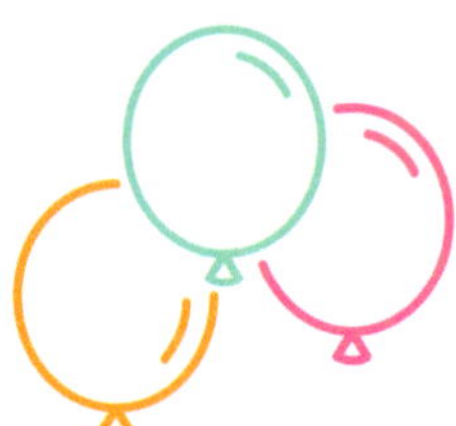
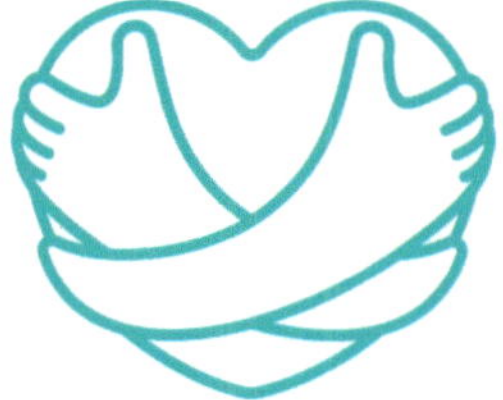
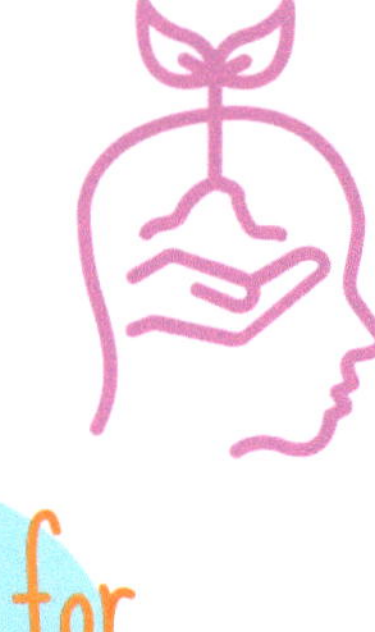
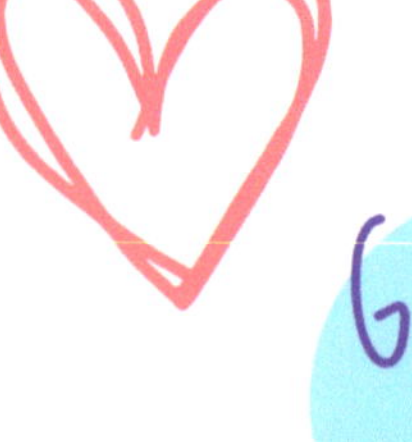
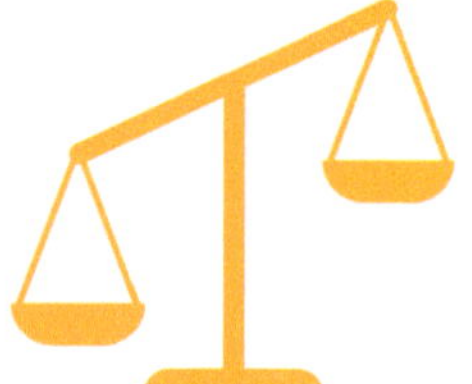
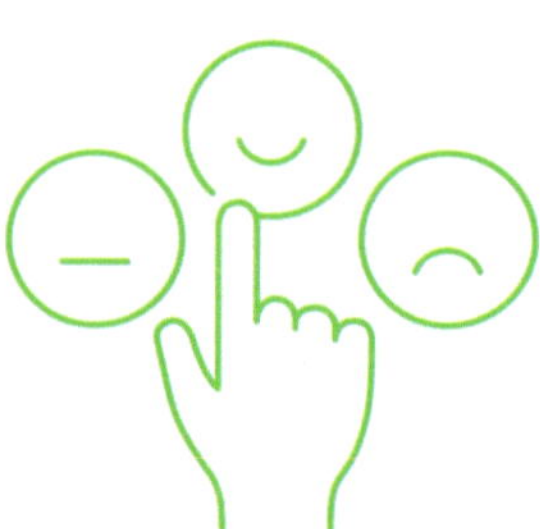
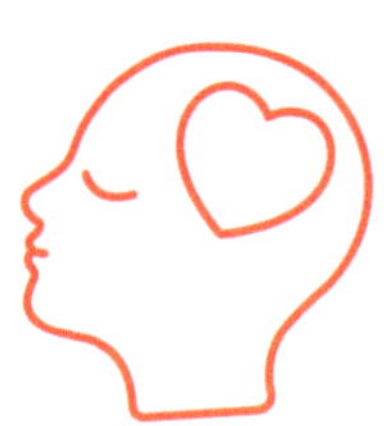

What's so great about YOGA?
Boosts self-esteem
It's so much fun
Great for mindfulness
Good for your heart
Strength and flexibility
Balance and coordination
Emotional regulation
Concentration and memory

"WHAT DO I NEED?"

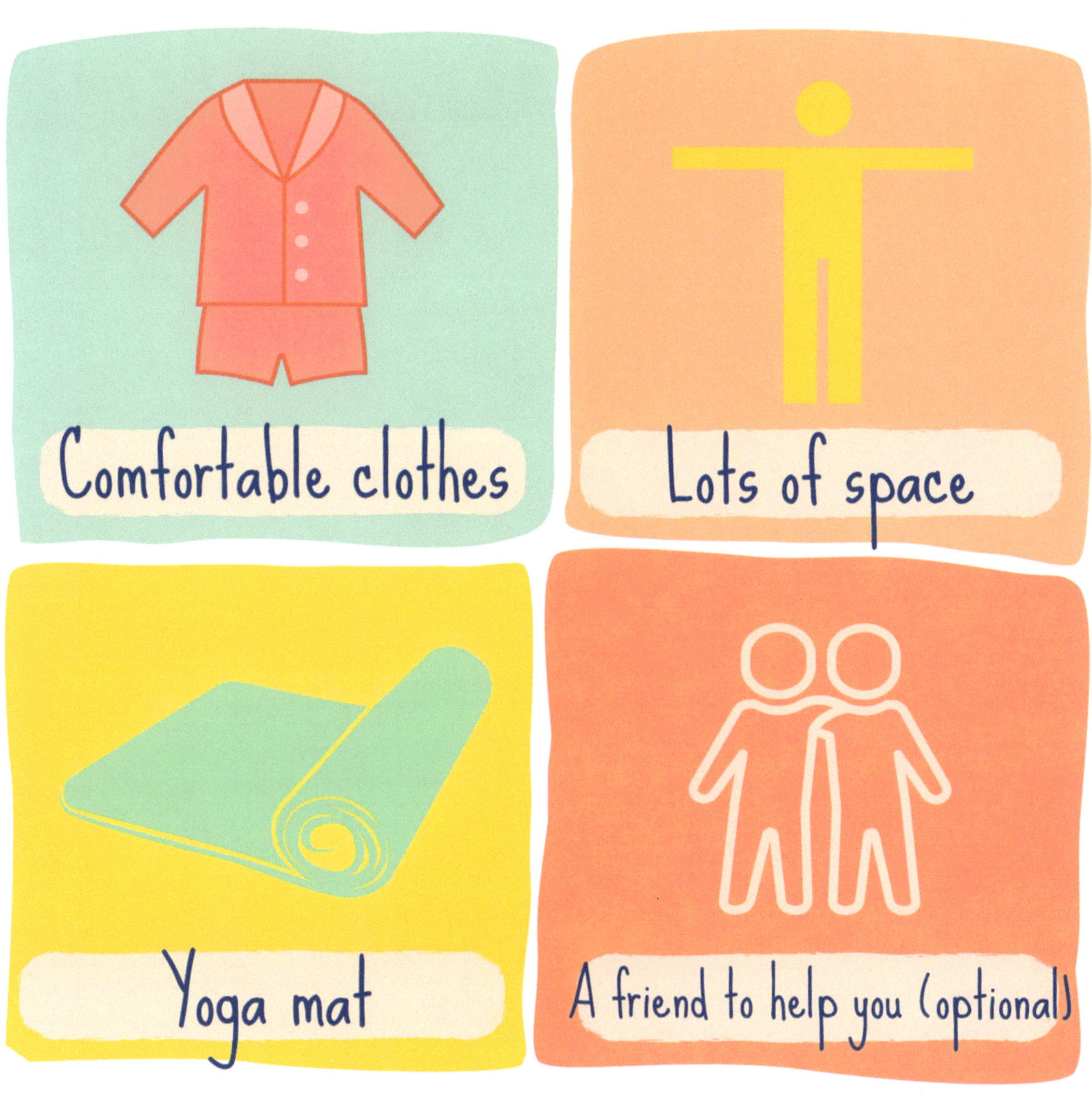

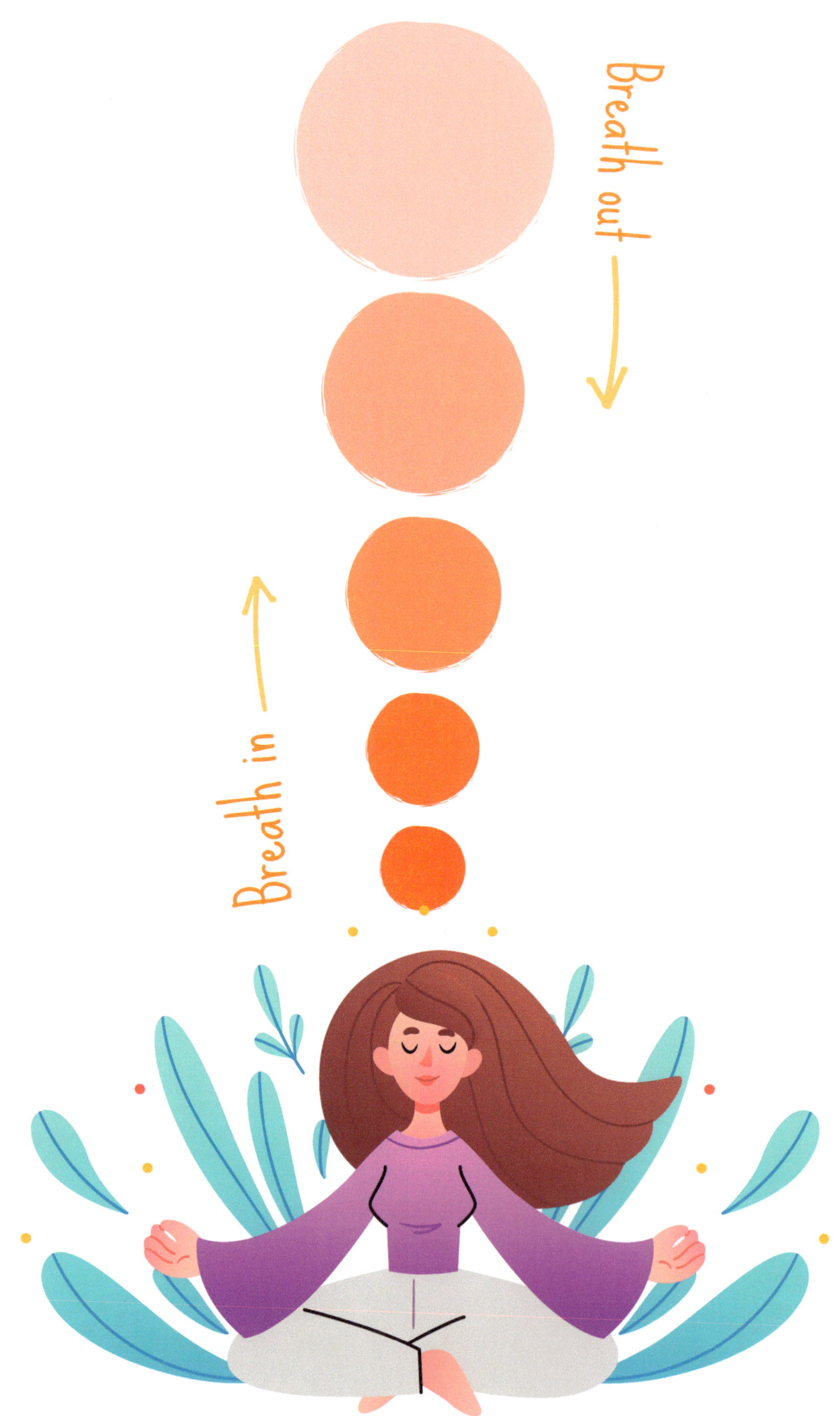
Breath out
Breath in

LET'S KICK OFF WITH SOME

Belly Breathing

1

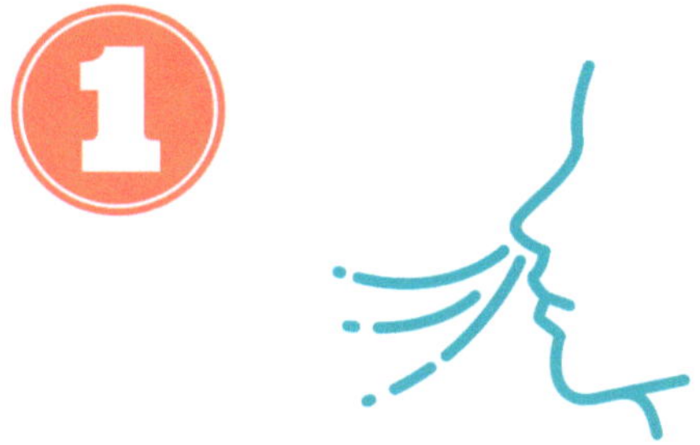

Take a deep breath in through your nose.

2

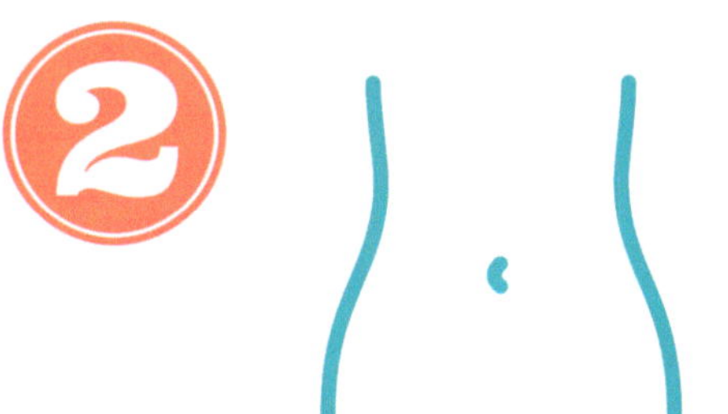

Fill your belly with your breath.

3

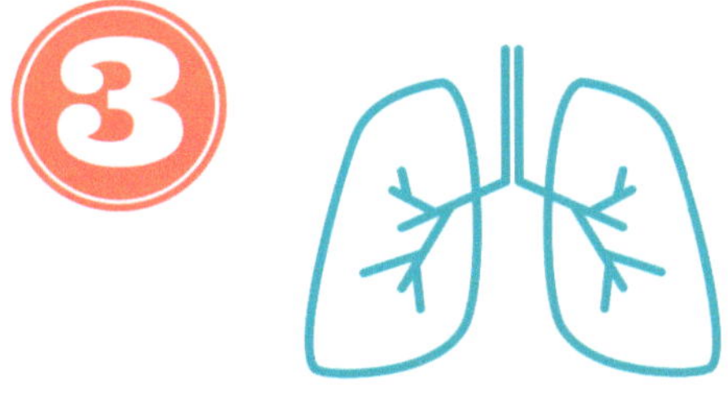

Continue to draw the breath in until it fills your lungs.

4

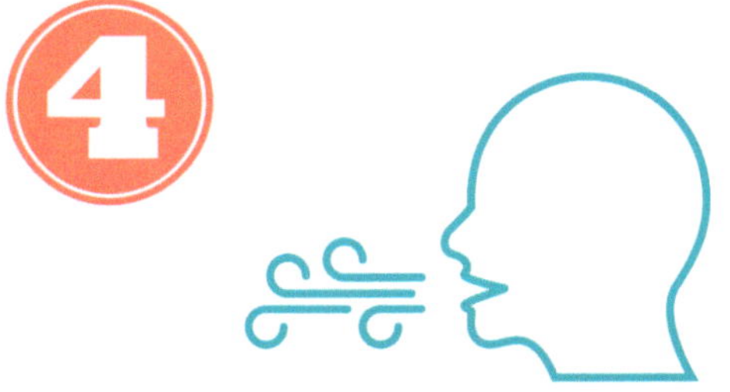

Slowly blow your breath out through your mouth.

What do you call a crazy space traveller?

What?

Astro-NUT

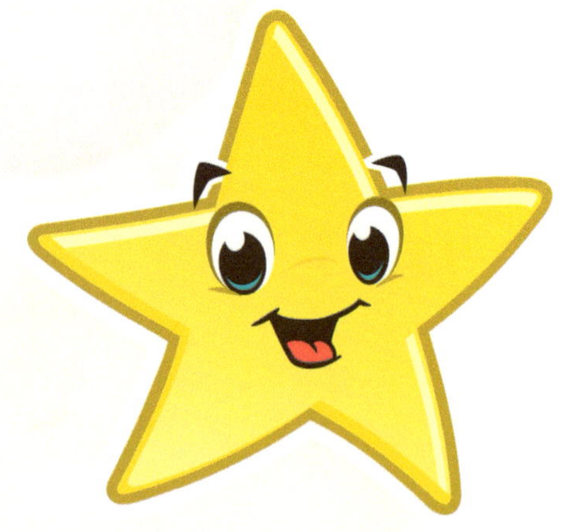

You say:
"I AM A STAR"

WOW!!!

WELL Done

TIP:
Try to touch the walls on either side of the room!

YOU GOT THIS!

Imagine this:
Your whole body starts to shine like a star. Your energy fills the room.

You can face your palms towards the floor, forward or up to the ceiling. YOU choose.

Stretched out arms

YAY

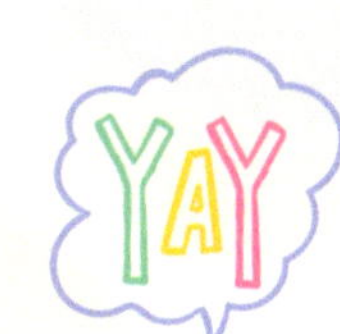

CHALLENGE:
Can you hold this pose for 10 seconds?

Stand up tall

You are doing GREAT!

Yoga mat (or just the floor)

GOOD JOB

Feet wide apart to where you feel comfort and balanced.

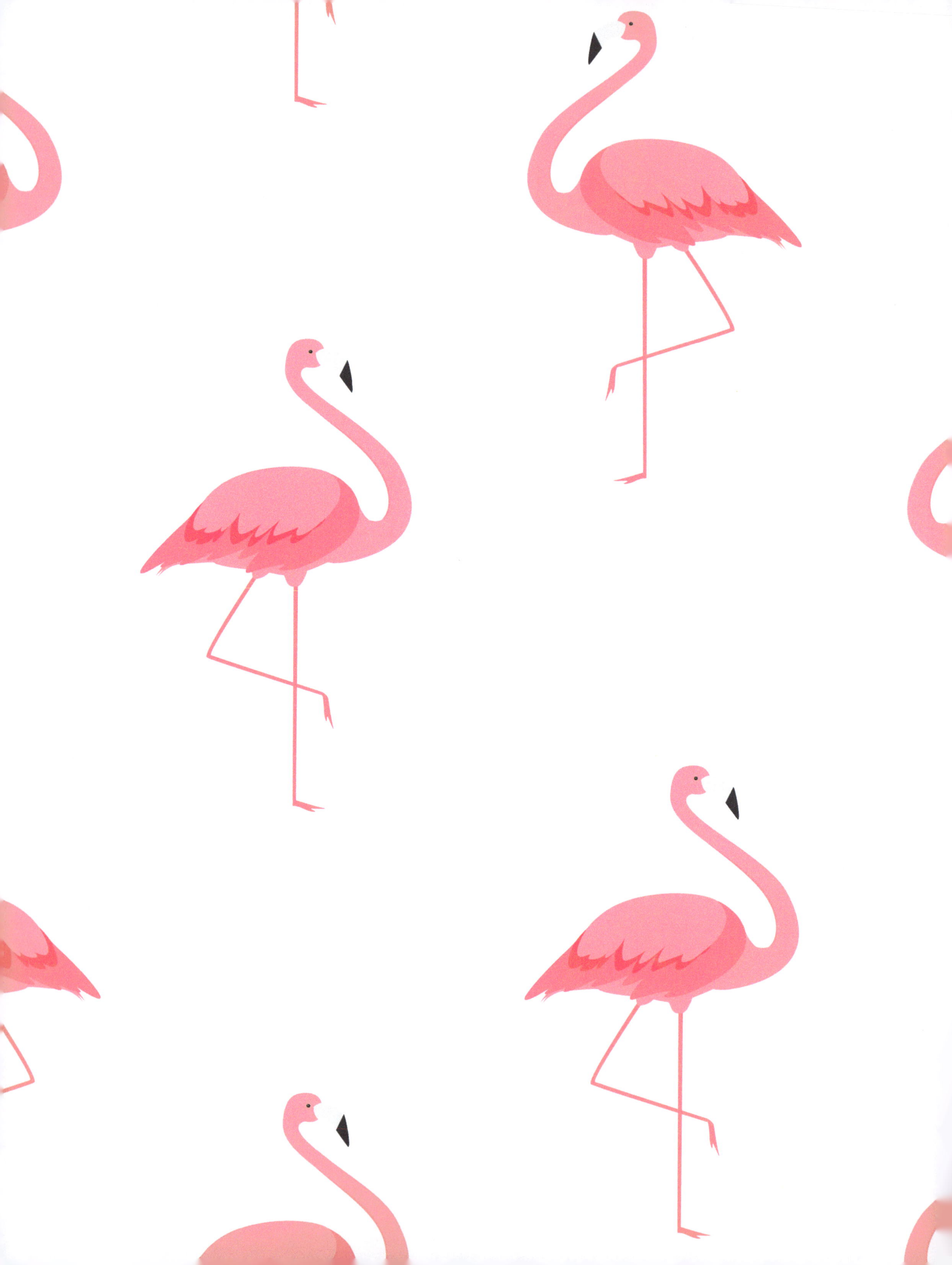

You say:
"I AM A FLAMINGO"

YAY!

Join your hands together over your head.

WOW!

CHALLENGE:
Can you balance in this pose for 5 seconds?

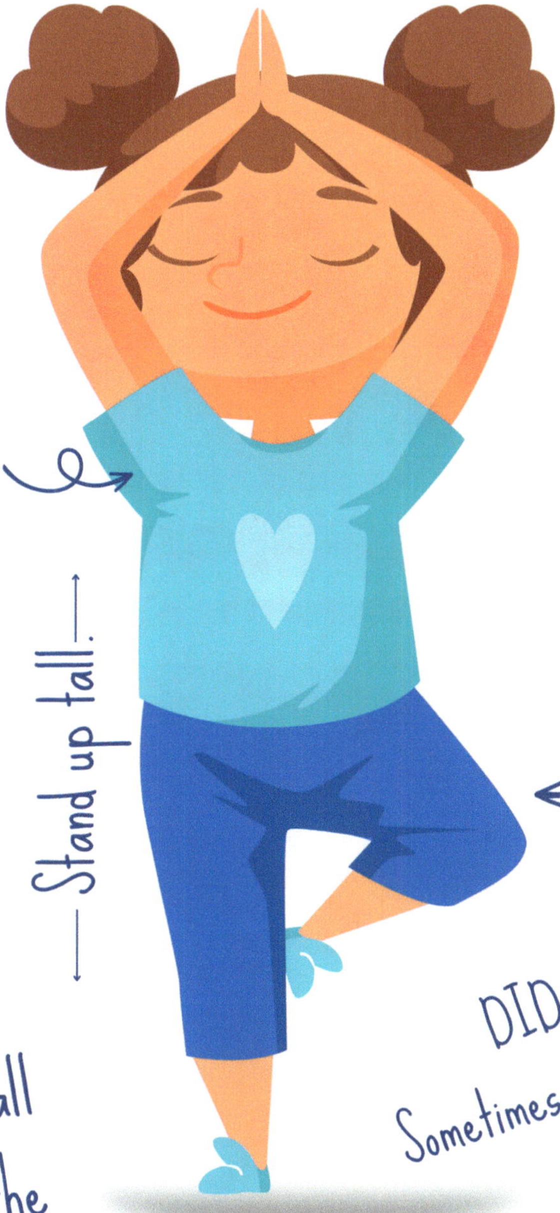

Bend your elbows.

Shoulders away from your ears.

Place the sole of your foot on your inner thigh of the standing leg.

Stand up tall.

GREAT BALANCE!.

Stand evenly on all four corners of the standing foot.

DID YOU KNOW?
Sometimes this move is called the TREE pose.

WOOHOO!

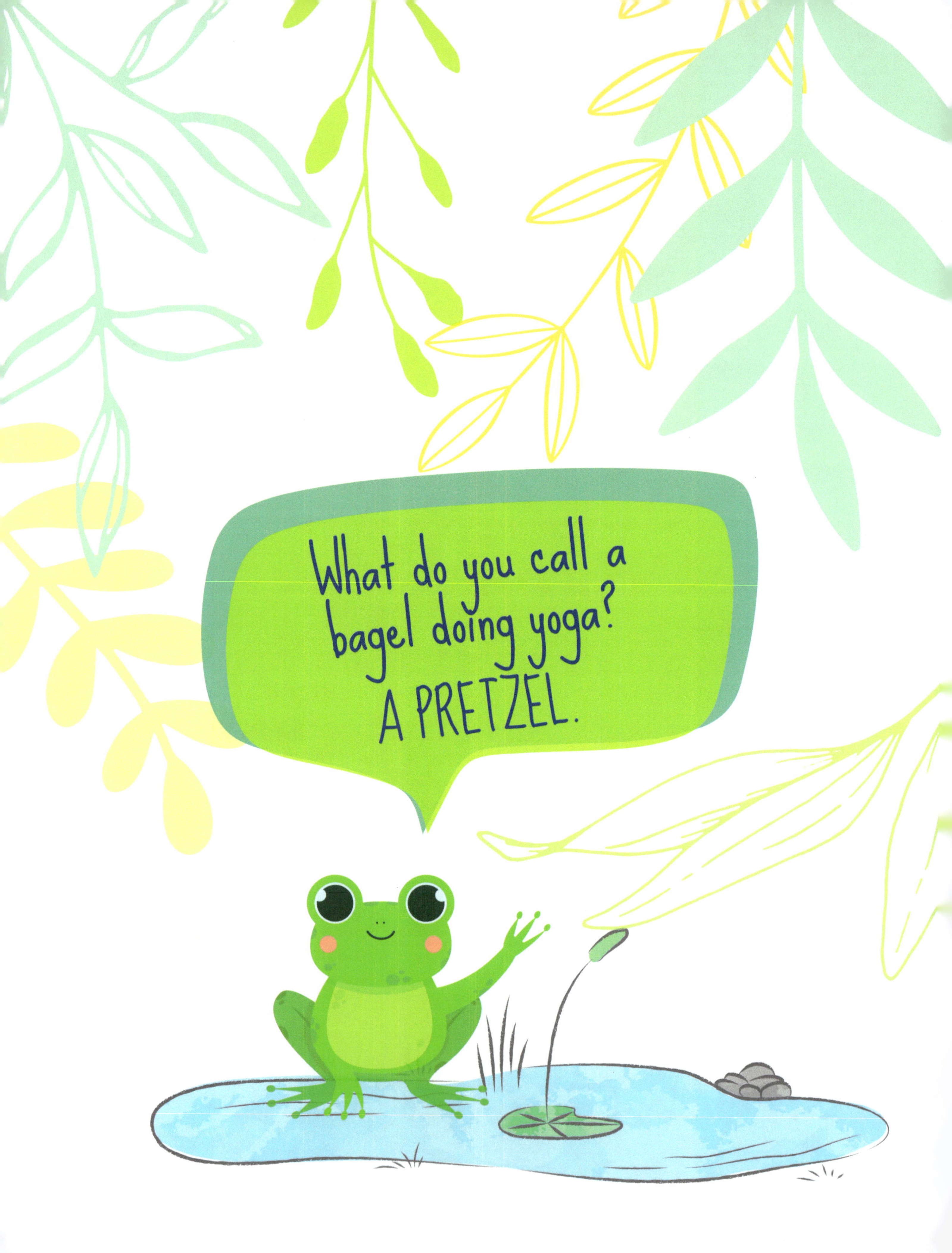

What do you call a bagel doing yoga?
A PRETZEL.

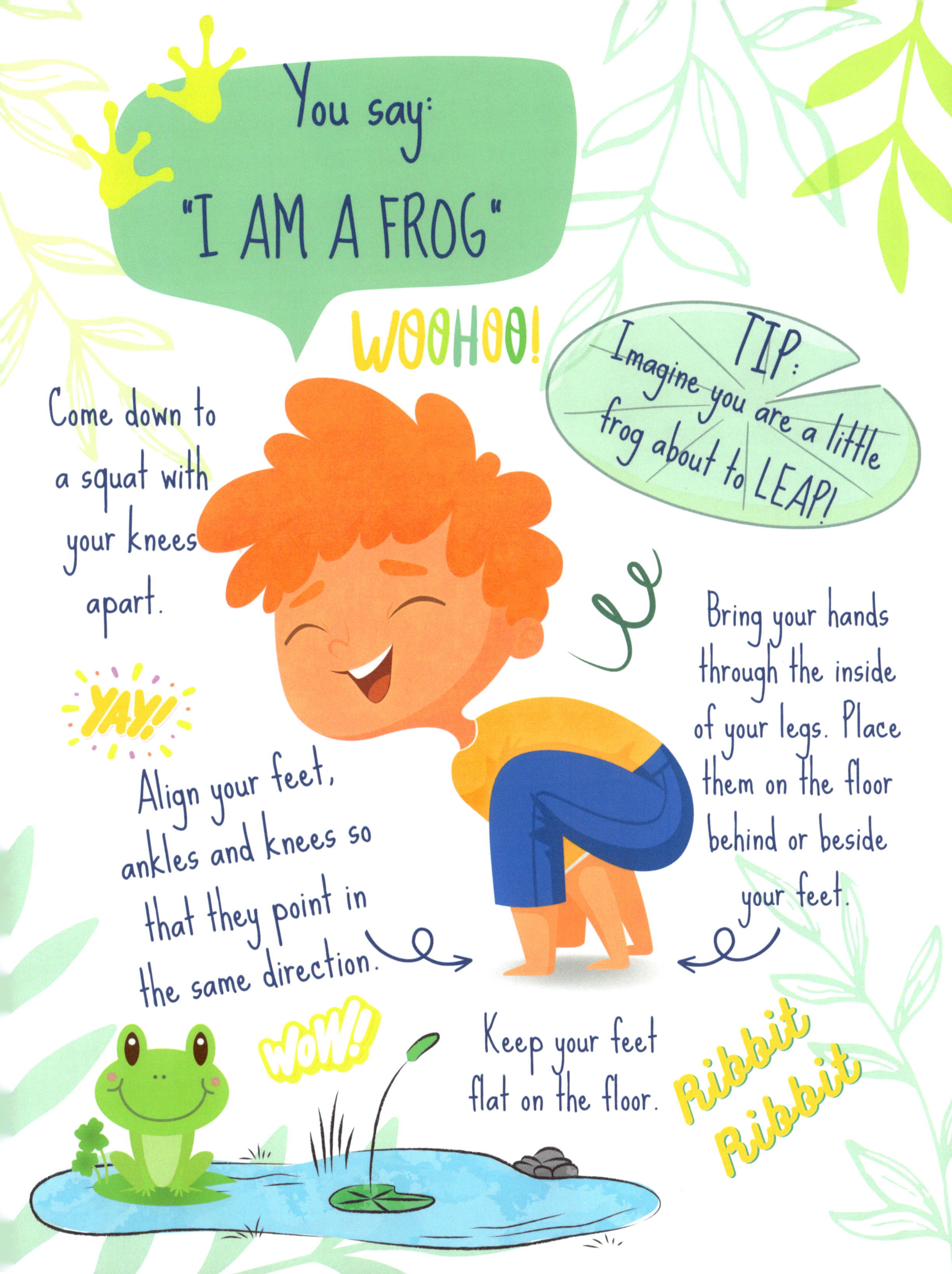

You say:
"I AM A FROG"
WOOHOO!
TIP:
Imagine you are a little frog about to LEAP!
Come down to a squat with your knees apart.
YAY!
Align your feet, ankles and knees so that they point in the same direction.
WOW!
Bring your hands through the inside of your legs. Place them on the floor behind or beside your feet.
Keep your feet flat on the floor.
Ribbit Ribbit

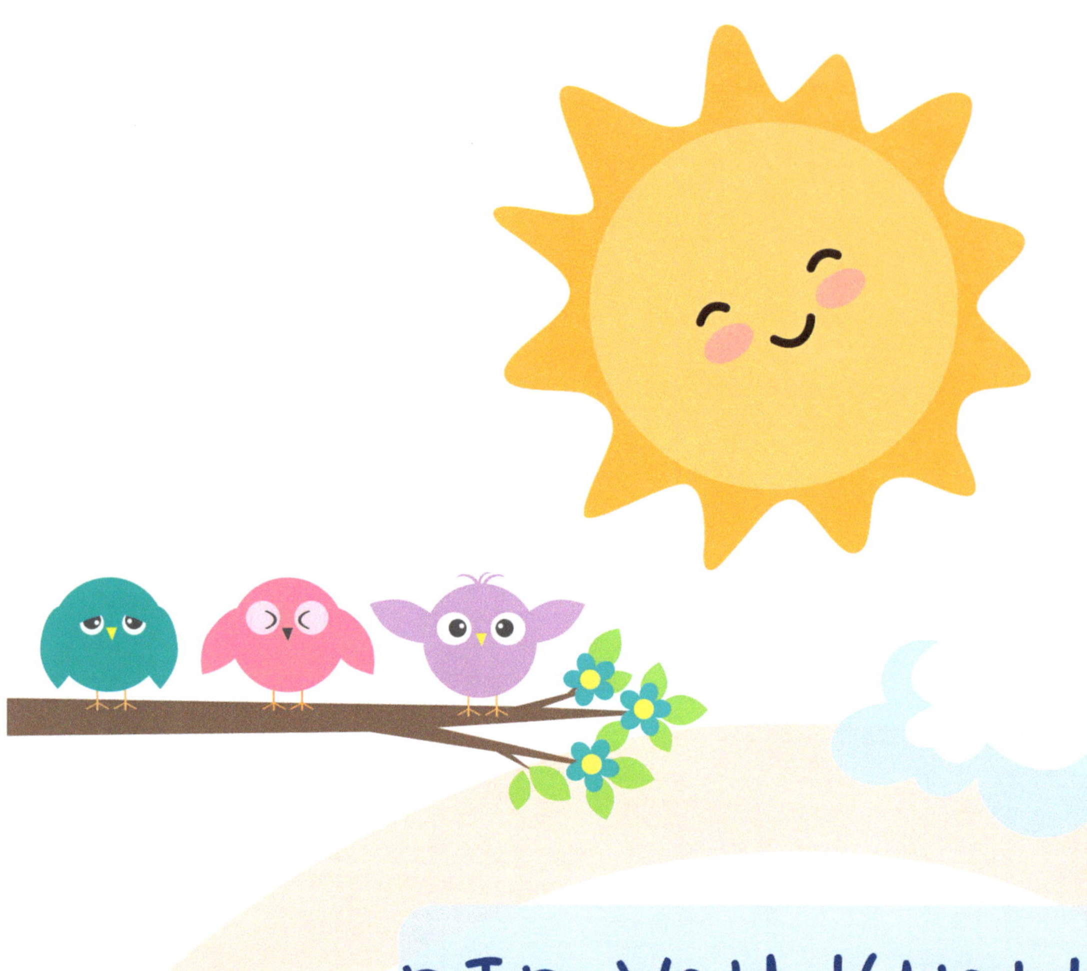
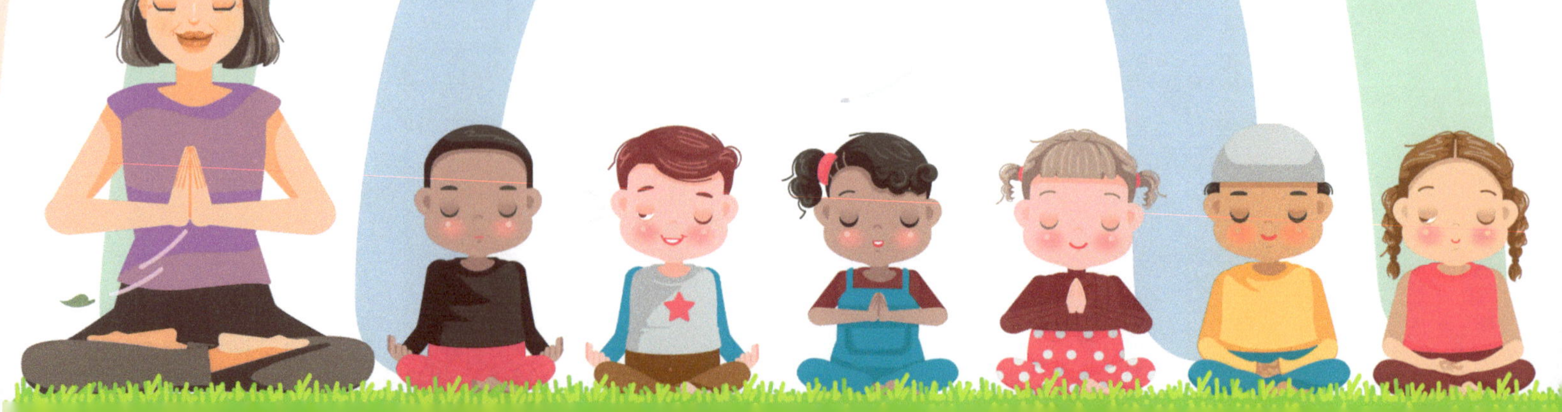

DID YOU KNOW?
Yoga is over 5000 years old.

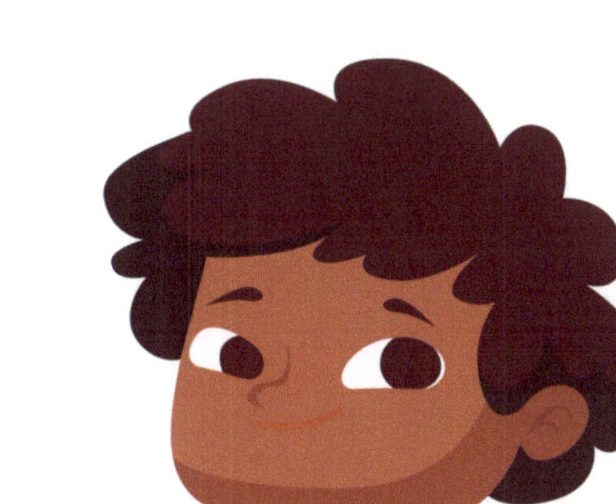

LIKE THE WARRIOR POSE?
Give this one a go too.

You say:
"I AM A WARRIOR"

good job

Stretch both arms out wide.
(reach for the wall on either side of the room).

Keep your back as straight as you can.

YAY!

Arms in line with shoulder.

Align your knee above your foot

Straight leg.

Point these toes to the front.

Point these toes to the side.

Keep those feet flat on the floor.

POWER

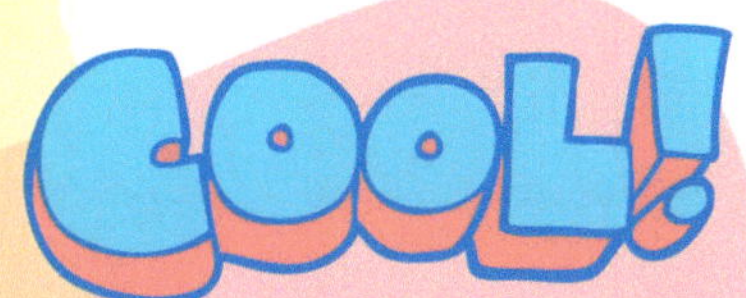

COOL!

Yoga... is...my... favourite....type... of... exercise.

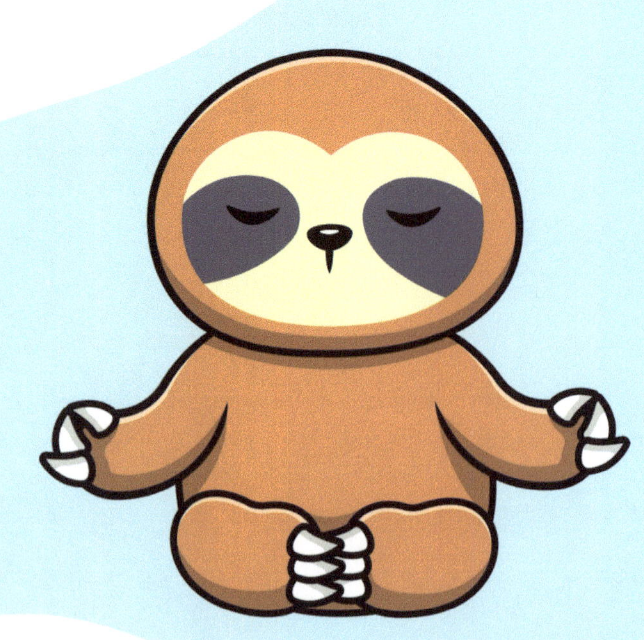

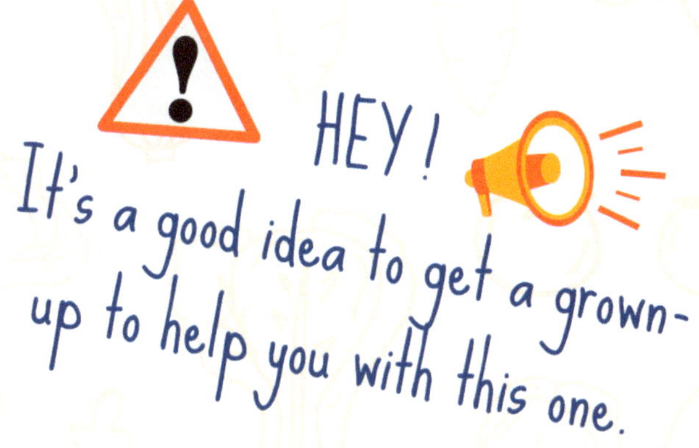

HEY!
It's a good idea to get a grown-up to help you with this one.

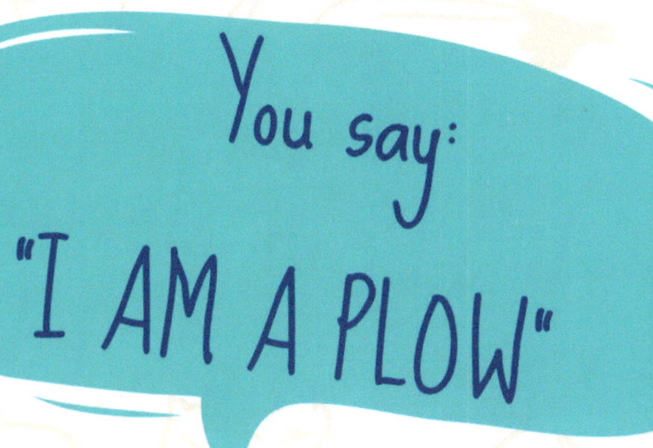

You say:
"I AM A PLOW"

TIP:
Imagine your trying to reach the sky with your bottom.

Shoot your tailbone upward towards the ceiling.

Unbend your knees

Do your feet reach the floor behind your head? GREAT! Press your toes into the ground.

Keep a straight back.

Press palms and fingers firmly into the floor.

Grab yourself a mat for your head.
(or something firm but soft to support you).

Look up at your knees. Don't twist your head!

YAY!

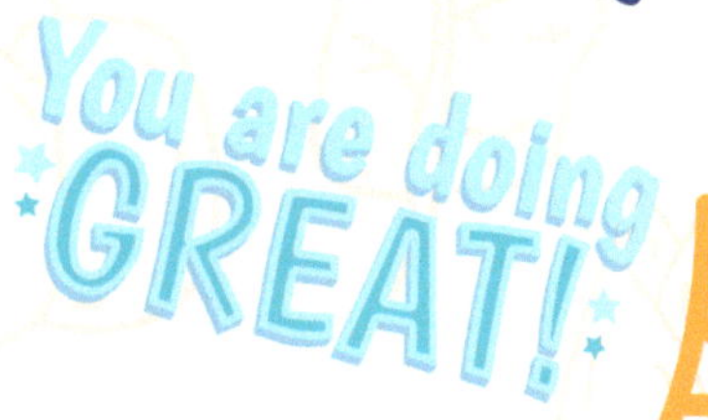

You are doing GREAT!

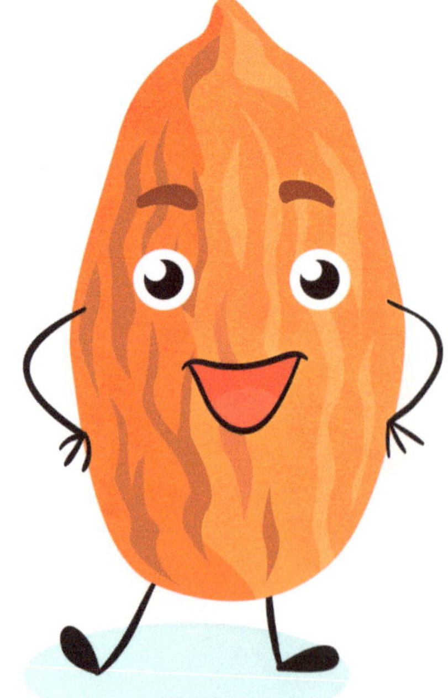
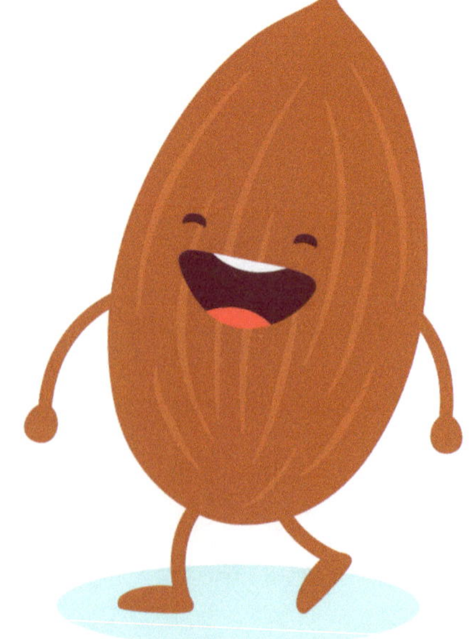
What's an elephant's favourite vegetable?
What?
SQUASH!

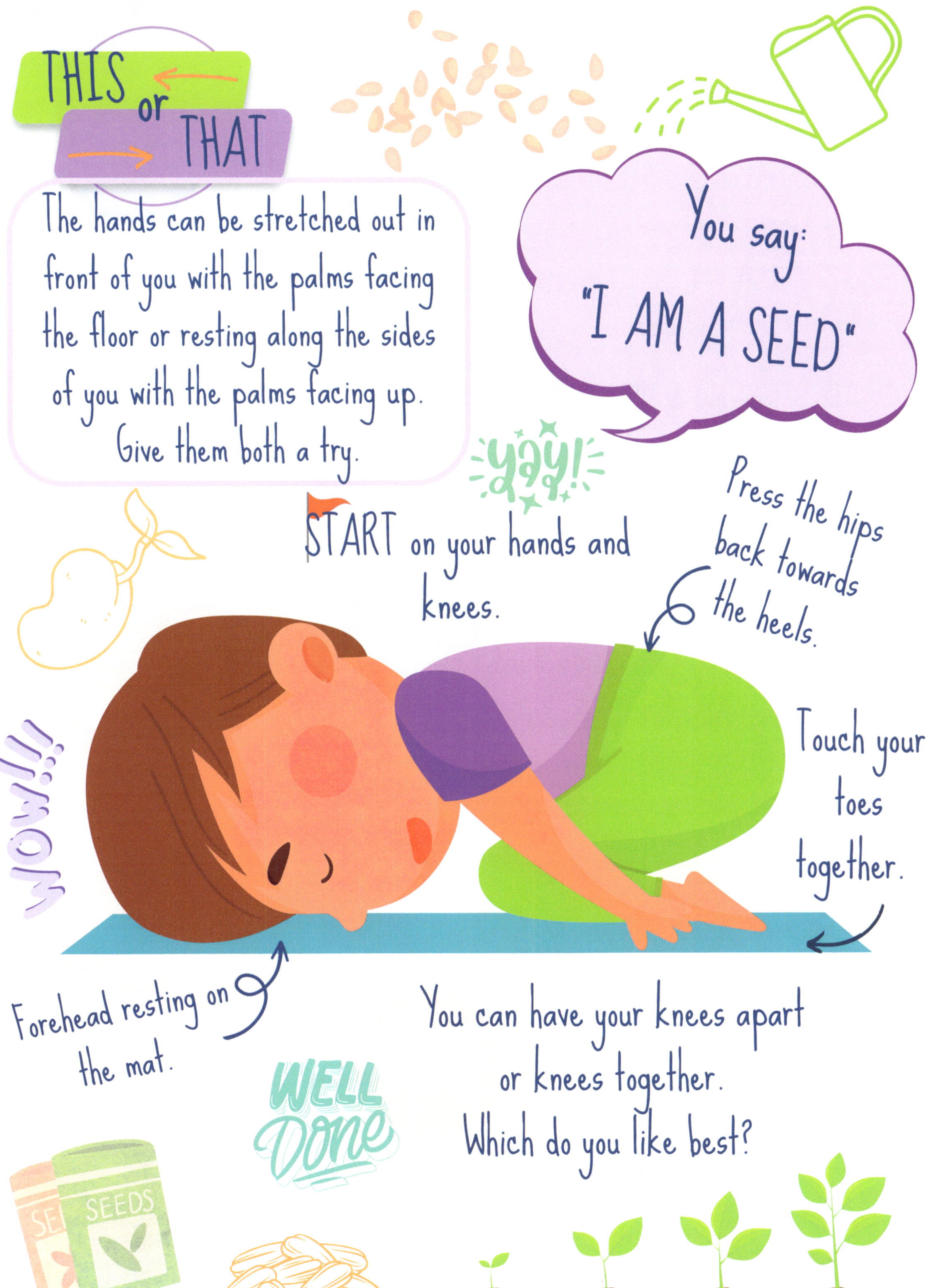

THIS or THAT
The hands can be stretched out in front of you with the palms facing the floor or resting along the sides of you with the palms facing up. Give them both a try.
You say: "I AM A SEED"
yay!
START on your hands and knees.
Press the hips back towards the heels.
WOW!!!
Touch your toes together.
Forehead resting on the mat.
WELL DONE
You can have your knees apart or knees together. Which do you like best?
SEEDS

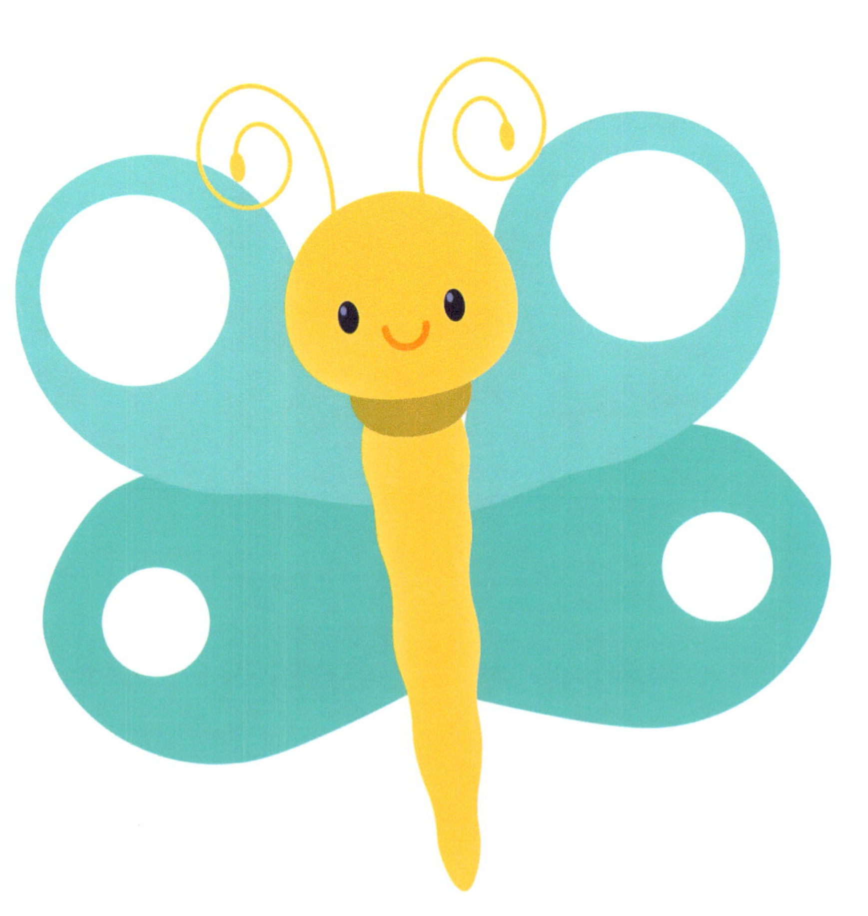

What happens when you throw a piece of butter out the window?
BUTTERFLY.

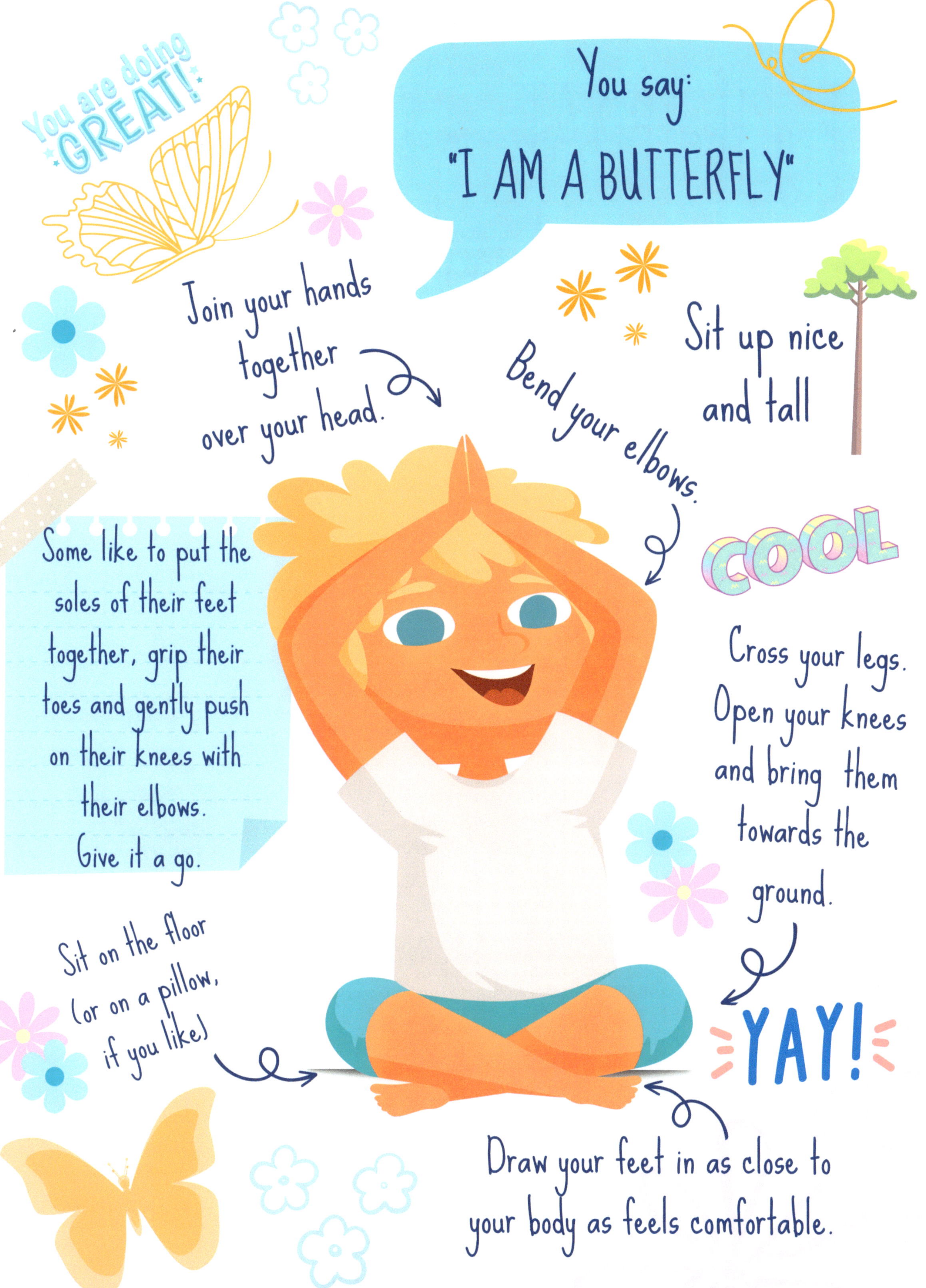

You are doing GREAT!
You say: "I AM A BUTTERFLY"
Join your hands together over your head.
Bend your elbows.
Sit up nice and tall
COOL
Some like to put the soles of their feet together, grip their toes and gently push on their knees with their elbows. Give it a go.
Cross your legs. Open your knees and bring them towards the ground.
Sit on the floor (or on a pillow, if you like)
YAY!
Draw your feet in as close to your body as feels comfortable.

Try the BOAT pose with a friend and make it TWICE AS FUN!

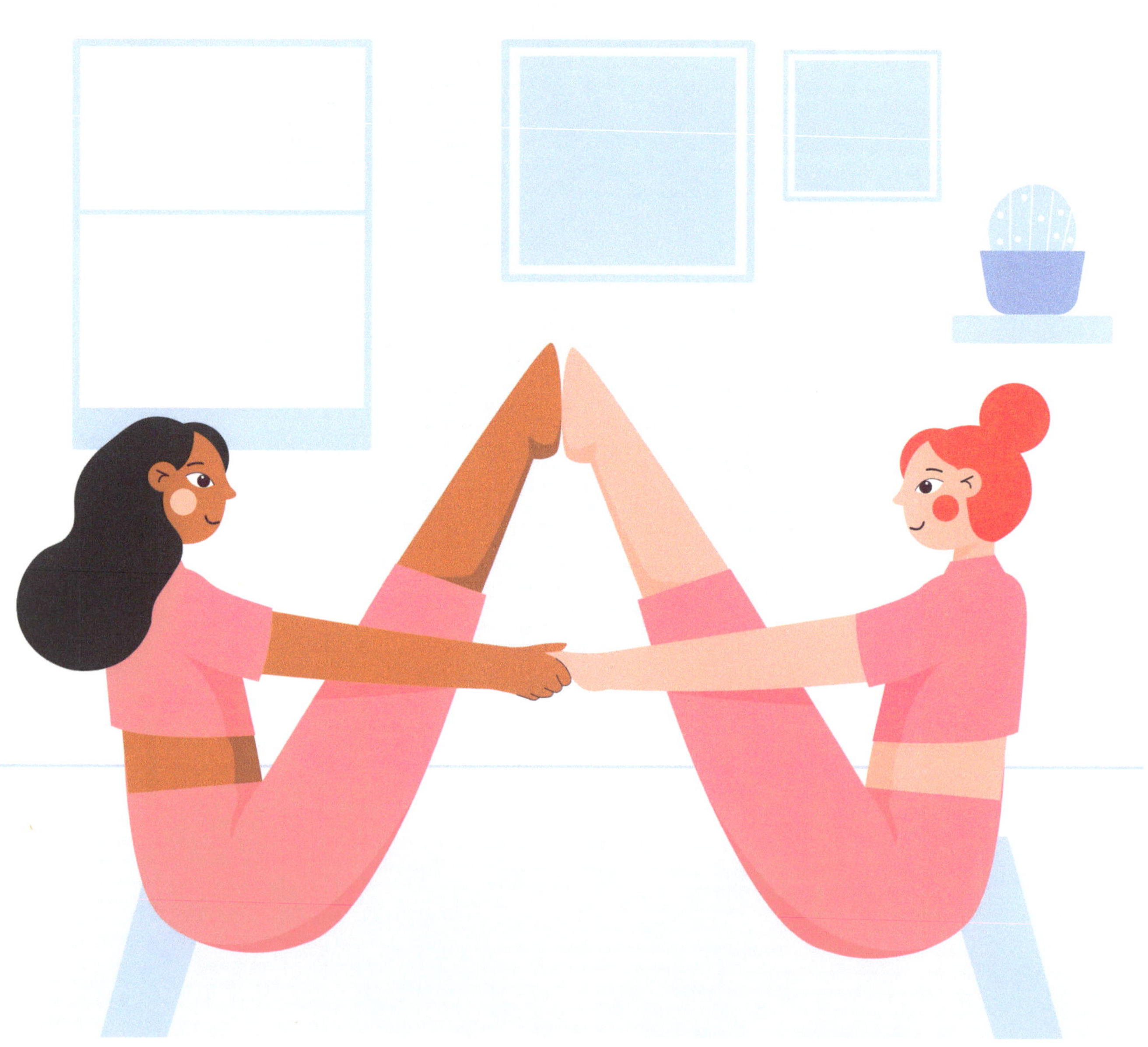

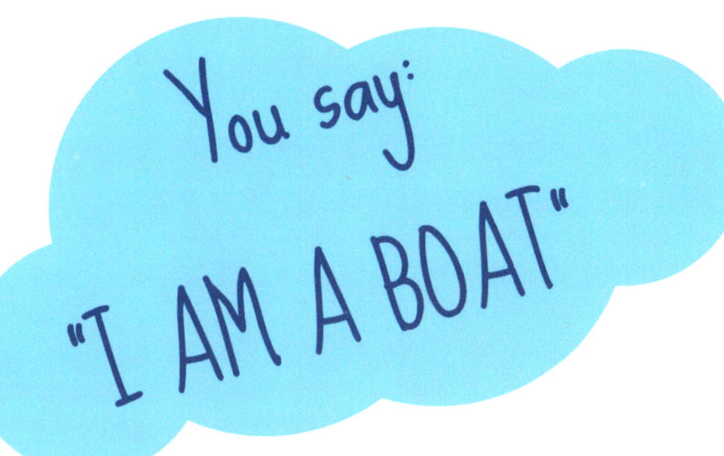

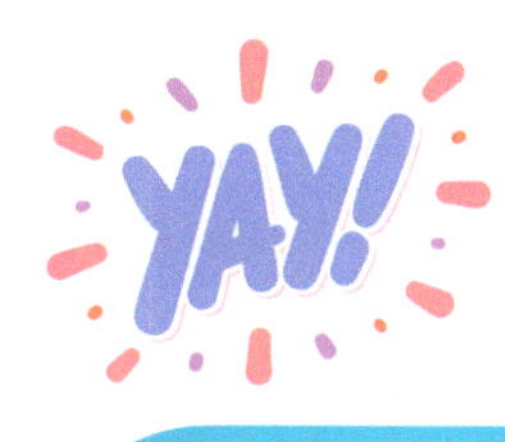

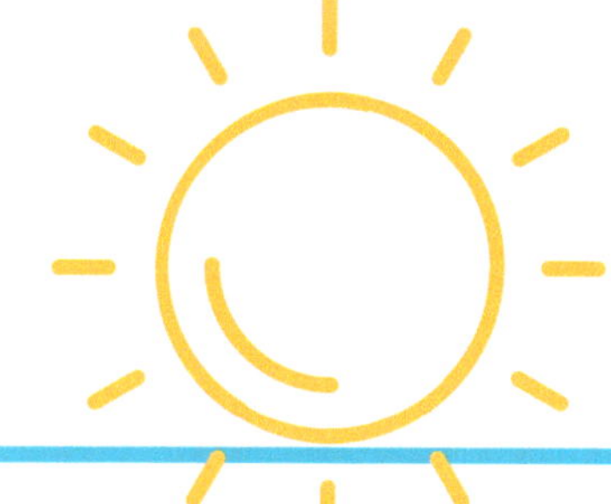

START - Lie down flat on your back with your hands by your side.
Reach for your toes with your arms.
Grasp your ankles if you can reach.

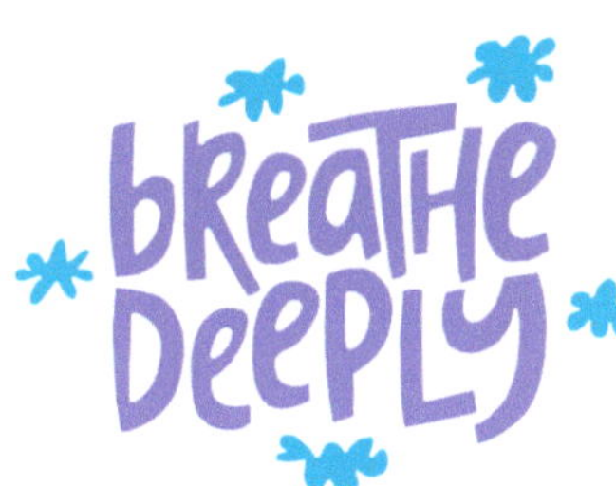

Lift your chest and feet off the ground to form a V shape.

Point your toes to the sky.

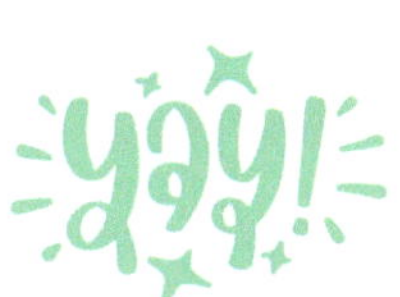

Keep those legs straight.

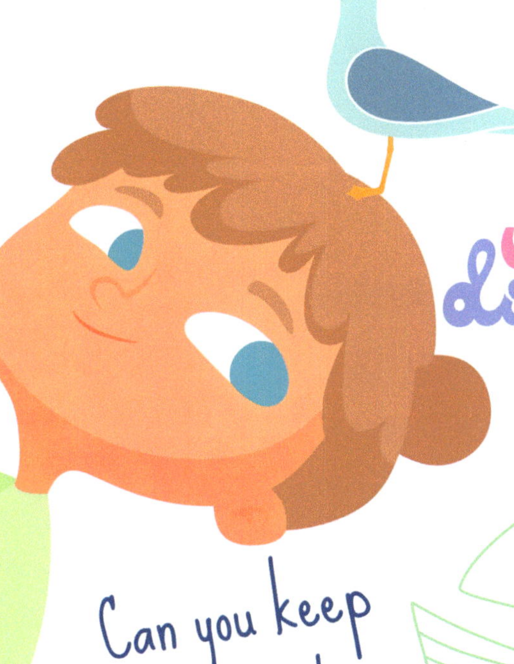

Can you keep your back straight?

Try to balance your weight on your bum.

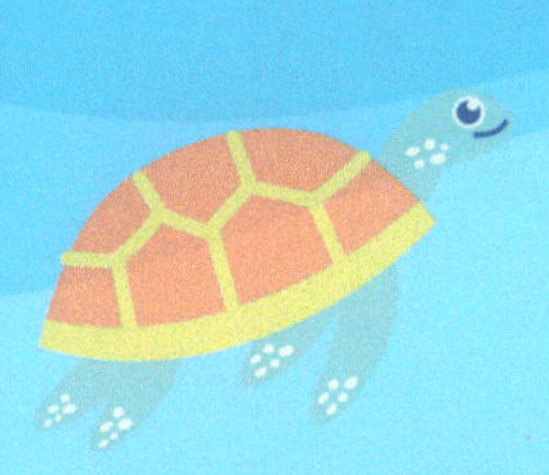
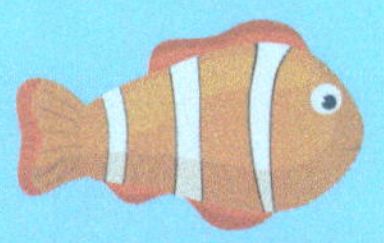
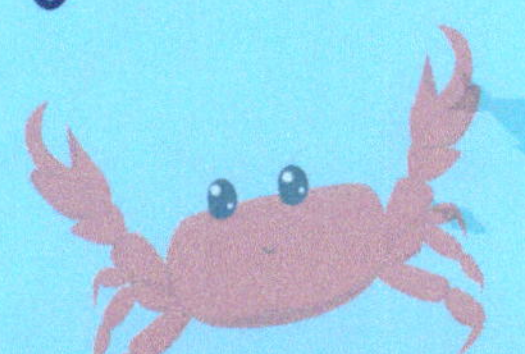
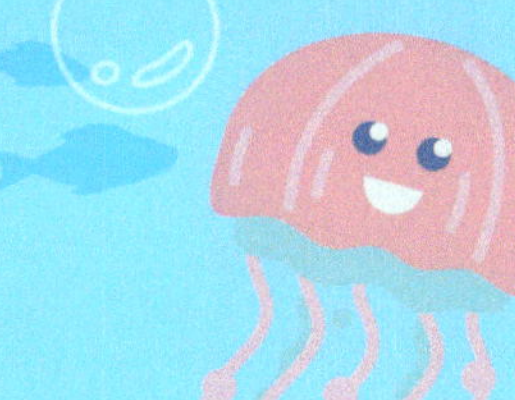
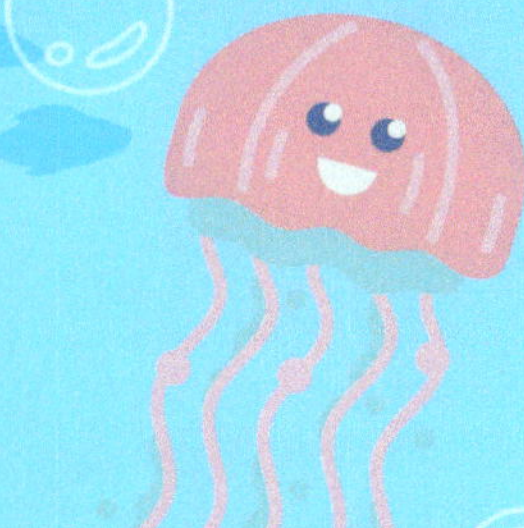

YOU DID IT
AWESOME
WOW!
2
1
3

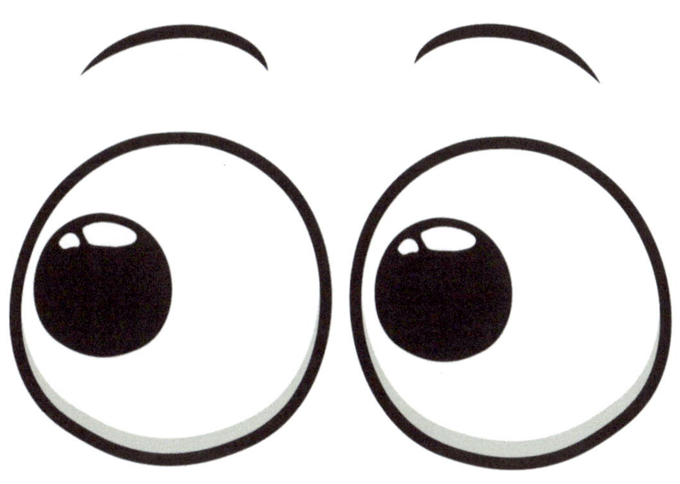

Pssst... Keep an eye out for

LITTLE YOGIS 2